Solutions and Prevention Against Mosquitoes, West Nile Virus, and More!

Buzzing Threats Revealed

Swift Health Solutionz Media

INTRODUCTION

CHAPTER 1

THE MIGHTY MOSQUITO: AN UNINVITED GUEST

THE LIFE CYCLE AND ANATOMY OF MOSQUITOES

DIFFERENT SPECIES OF MOSQUITOES AND THEIR GEOGRAPHICAL DISTRIBUTION

THE ECOLOGICAL IMPORTANCE OF MOSQUITOES AND THEIR ROLE AS DISEASE VECTORS

FACTORS CONTRIBUTING TO THE PROLIFERATION OF MOSQUITOES

CHAPTER 2

UNMASKING WEST NILE VIRUS: THE SILENT INTRUDER

THE BIOLOGY OF WEST NILE VIRUS AND ITS TRANSMISSION CYCLE

CLINICAL MANIFESTATIONS, DIAGNOSIS, AND TREATMENT OF WEST NILE VIRUS INFECTION

IMPACT OF WEST NILE VIRUS ON PUBLIC HEALTH, ECONOMICS, AND AFFECTED COMMUNITIES

CHAPTER 3

BATTLING MOSQUITO-BORNE DISEASES: PREVENTION AND CONTROL

PREVENTING AND CONTROLLING MOSQUITO-BORNE DISEASES, INCLUDING WEST NILE VIRUS

PERSONAL PROTECTIVE MEASURES FOR MOSQUITO-BORNE DISEASES

COMMUNITY-BASED INTERVENTIONS FOR MOSQUITO CONTROL AND PUBLIC AWARENESS

THE ROLE OF TECHNOLOGY AND INNOVATION IN MOSQUITO CONTROL

CHAPTER 4

THE FUTURE OF MOSQUITO-BORNE DISEASE MANAGEMENT

CURRENT ADVANCEMENTS IN MOSQUITO CONTROL AND DISEASE MANAGEMENT

Challenges and Opportunities in the Fight Against Mosquito-Borne Diseases

The Potential of Emerging Technologies in Disease Prevention and Control

CONCLUSION

INTRODUCTION

In today's interconnected world, infectious disease threats loom large, sparking growing global concern. From the devastating impact of pandemics like COVID-19 to the persistent threat of mosquito-borne illnesses, the need for a comprehensive understanding of these diseases and effective prevention measures has never been more crucial. Among the myriad disease-transmitting culprits, mosquitoes take center stage as notorious vectors responsible for spreading various dangerous infections. This book delves into the intricate relationship between mosquitoes, the West Nile virus, and infectious diseases, exploring their causes, solutions, prevention strategies, and modes of transmission.

This book's heart lies in the significance of the West Nile virus, one of the most prominent and pernicious mosquito-borne diseases. This virulent pathogen has wreaked havoc on human health across the globe, affecting millions and leaving a trail of illness and even death in its wake. The impact of the West Nile virus is far-reaching, striking fear in communities and straining healthcare systems worldwide. By understanding the complexities of this disease, we can unlock the potential for effective prevention and control measures to mitigate its devastating consequences.

The book is organized into five chapters, each dedicated to unraveling different aspects of mosquito menace and infectious diseases. In Chapter 1, "The Mighty Mosquito: An Uninvited Guest," we embark on a journey into the world of mosquitoes, understanding their life cycle, diverse species, and ecological significance. We uncover the factors that contribute to their proliferation, including the influence of climate change and urbanization.

Chapter 2, "Unmasking West Nile Virus: The Silent Intruder," sheds light on the origins and history of the West Nile virus, tracing its discovery, initial outbreaks, and global spread. We delve into the biology of the virus, examining its transmission cycle between mosquitoes, birds, and humans. The chapter also explores West Nile virus infection's clinical manifestations, diagnostic methods, and available treatment options.

In Chapter 3, "Battling Mosquito-Borne Diseases: Prevention and Control," we navigate the realm of prevention strategies for mosquito-borne diseases, specifically focusing on the West Nile virus. We discuss personal protective measures such as insect repellents, protective clothing, bed nets, and community-based interventions like mosquito control programs and public awareness campaigns. Additionally, we explore the role of technology and innovation in mosquito control, including genetically modified mosquitoes and novel insecticides.

Chapter 4, "Beyond West Nile: Other Mosquito-Borne Diseases," widens our lens to encompass other significant mosquito-borne diseases such as dengue fever, Zika virus, malaria, and Chikungunya. We provide a comprehensive overview of each condition, detailing its causes, symptoms, geographical distribution, and impact on public health. By comparing these diseases to the West Nile virus, we gain valuable insights into the similarities and differences, enhancing our understanding of the broader mosquito-borne disease landscape.

Finally, in Chapter 5, "The Future of Mosquito-Borne Disease Management," we peer into the crystal ball of disease management. We explore cutting-edge advancements in mosquito control, disease surveillance, and treatment options. The chapter discusses the challenges and opportunities in combating mosquito-borne diseases, considering climate change, drug resistance, and international cooperation. Moreover, we contemplate the potential of emerging technologies like gene editing and predictive modeling in revolutionizing disease prevention and control.

With this book, we aim to empower readers with knowledge and insights to combat the threat of mosquito-borne diseases. By understanding the causes, solutions, prevention strategies, and modes of transmission, we can collectively work towards a future where the buzzing threats of mosquitoes are effectively neutralized and infectious diseases are relegated to the annals of history. Let us embark

On this illuminating journey together, safeguarding our health and well-being.

CHAPTER 1
The Mighty Mosquito: An Uninvited Guest

The Life Cycle and Anatomy of Mosquitoes

Mosquitoes, those tiny buzzing creatures that seem to have an uncanny ability to find us at the most inconvenient times, are far more than mere nuisances. To understand their role as vectors for transmitting infectious diseases, it is crucial to explore their fascinating life cycle and intricate anatomy, which enable them to thrive and adapt in various environments.

The life cycle of a mosquito consists of four distinct stages: egg, larva, pupa, and adult. It begins with the female mosquito laying her eggs on the surface of stagnant water or in areas prone to flooding. These eggs, resembling tiny black dots, can be found in clusters or individually, depending on the species. Interestingly, some mosquito species lay their eggs in a manner that allows them to withstand desiccation, ensuring their survival even in unfavorable conditions.

Once the eggs come into contact with water, they hatch into larvae, commonly known as "wrigglers." These wrigglers are aquatic creatures equipped with unique adaptations to thrive in water. They possess a slender, elongated body with a different head and a series of bristle-like appendages called siphons. These siphons, located at the posterior end of the larvae, enable them to access air at the water's surface for breathing.

The larval stage is marked by rapid growth and molting as the larvae feed voraciously on microorganisms, algae, and organic matter in the water. Their diet is vital to their development, ensuring they accumulate the necessary energy and nutrients to progress to the next stage. During this period, the larvae undergo several molts, shedding their exoskeleton to accommodate their increasing size.

After several molts, the larvae enter the pupal stage, a transformative period in their life cycle. Pupae are comma-shaped and distinctly different from the larvae. They possess respiratory trumpets acting as breathing tubes, allowing them to obtain oxygen from the surrounding water. Pupae do not actively feed but rely on the energy reserves accumulated during their larval stage. Inside the pupal case, profound changes occur as the larval tissues undergo a remarkable metamorphosis, gradually transforming into adult structures.

Finally, the pupal case splits open, and the adult mosquito emerges, ready to take flight into the world. The adult mosquito is characterized by its familiar, delicate, slender body adorned with long, segmented antennae. The most distinguishing feature of the female mosquito is her mouthparts, specifically designed for piercing and sucking blood. Unlike males, which primarily feed on nectar and plant juices, females require a blood meal to obtain the necessary proteins for egg development.

While the life cycle of a mosquito is intriguing, it is their ability to adapt to diverse environments that truly sets them apart. Mosquitoes have evolved to occupy many habitats, from tropical rainforests to arid desert regions. They have even adapted to urban environments, thriving amidst the concrete jungles of bustling cities. This adaptability is partly due to their genetic plasticity, allowing them to adjust their physiological and behavioral characteristics to match their surroundings.

Furthermore, mosquitoes are incredibly resilient creatures. They possess a remarkable ability to survive in adverse conditions, including extreme temperatures and limited resources. Certain mosquito species can enter diapause or dormancy during unfavorable seasons or when resources are scarce. This allows them to survive droughts, cold winters, or other environmental challenges until favorable conditions return.

The anatomy of mosquitoes is also finely tuned for their survival and success as disease vectors. The female mosquito's mouthparts comprise a complex structure known as the proboscis, which includes multiple.

Components designed to facilitate efficient blood-feeding. These include a pair of mandibles and maxillae that pierce the skin, while a labrum acts as a sheath to protect the delicate parts during feeding. The mosquito's saliva, injected into the host during feeding, contains anticoagulant compounds that prevent the blood from clotting and facilitate a continuous flow of the mosquito's meal.

In addition to their unique feeding apparatus, mosquitoes possess a unique sensory system. Their long antennae, covered in tiny hairs, are sensitive receptors for detecting carbon dioxide, heat, moisture, and chemical cues emitted by potential hosts. This remarkable sense of smell enables them to quickly track down their victims, often from a considerable distance.

As our understanding of mosquito biology and anatomy deepens, so does our ability to devise effective prevention and control strategies. By comprehending their life cycle, adaptive traits, and remarkable anatomical features, we gain insights into their vulnerabilities and identify potential targets for intervention. With this knowledge, researchers, public health officials, and communities can work hand in hand to combat the menace of mosquitoes and the infectious diseases they carry.

Different Species of Mosquitoes and Their Geographical Distribution

Mosquitoes, the uninvited guests that relentlessly buzz around us, come in various species, each with its own ecological niche and geographical distribution. While not all mosquitoes transmit diseases, several species have gained notoriety as vectors of deadly infections. Understanding mosquito species' diversity and distribution is essential for effective disease surveillance, prevention, and control efforts.

There are approximately 3,500 known species of mosquitoes worldwide belonging to the family Culicidae. However, not all species are involved in disease transmission. It is primarily the female mosquitoes that feed on blood, requiring it for egg development. Thus, it is the female mosquitoes that pose the most significant risk as disease vectors.

Among the most well-known disease-transmitting mosquitoes are the genus Anopheles, Aedes, and Culex members. Anopheles mosquitoes are infamous for transmitting malaria, a parasitic disease that affects millions of people globally, particularly in sub-Saharan Africa, Southeast Asia, and parts of Latin America. The Anopheles genus comprises numerous species, each with a preference for particular environmental conditions, such as stagnant water bodies or flowing streams.

Aedes mosquitoes have gained significant attention recently due to their role in transmitting diseases like dengue fever, Zika virus, and chikungunya. Aedes aegypti, in particular, is a primary vector for these diseases and is widely distributed in tropical and subtropical regions worldwide. This species thrives in urban environments, breeding in small water containers commonly found in and around human habitations.

On the other hand, Culex mosquitoes are known for transmitting diseases such as West Nile virus and Japanese encephalitis. Culex pipiens and Culex quinquefasciatus are two prominent species within this genus, with a global distribution. They are versatile mosquitoes, adapting well to various urban, suburban, and rural environments.

The geographical distribution of disease-transmitting mosquitoes is influenced by several factors, including climate, ecology, and human activities. For example, Anopheles mosquitoes, responsible for transmitting malaria, are most prevalent in tropical and subtropical regions with warm and humid climates. These areas provide ideal conditions for mosquito breeding and parasite development within the mosquito's body.

Aedes mosquitoes, which transmit dengue fever, Zika virus, and chikungunya, have a wider distribution and can be found in tropical, subtropical, and temperate regions. Their presence is influenced by factors such as temperature, rainfall, and the availability of breeding sites. With increasing globalization and travel, these mosquitoes have the potential to spread diseases to new regions, as seen in recent outbreaks of dengue and Zika in areas previously unaffected.

Culex mosquitoes, known for transmitting West Nile virus and Japanese encephalitis, have a broader geographical range, including tropical and temperate regions. Their adaptability allows them to breed in various water sources, from natural bodies of water to artificial containers like discarded tires and bird baths.

It is important to note that the distribution of disease-transmitting mosquitoes can change over time. Factors such as urbanization, deforestation, climate change, and human mobility can alter the habitat suitability for these mosquitoes, leading to shifts in their geographical range. Understanding these dynamics is crucial for anticipating and responding to the emergence or re-emergence of mosquito-borne diseases in different regions.

Efforts to combat mosquito-borne diseases involve targeting specific species and considering the ecological context in which they thrive. Integrated vector management strategies encompass a range of approaches, including mosquito control programs, elimination of breeding sites,

use of insecticides and community-based interventions. These strategies must be tailored to the unique characteristics of the target mosquito species and the local ecological conditions.

The Ecological Importance of Mosquitoes and Their Role as Disease Vectors

Mosquitoes, those humming irritations that unendingly irritate us, may appear to be a disturbance, yet they assume a critical part in different biological systems, showing a natural significance that reaches out past their status as sickness vectors. It is essential to comprehend the broader ecological context in which mosquitoes operate, despite the fact that we acknowledge their role in the transmission of infectious diseases.

The insect family known as Diptera includes mosquitoes, flies, and midges. They are an essential component of the food web because they provide numerous organisms with essential food. In aquatic habitats, mosquito larvae, also known as wrigglers, consume organic matter and microorganisms, assisting in the cycle of nutrients and preserving ecosystem equilibrium. Thus, the hatchlings act as prey for fish, creatures of land and water, reptiles, and insectivorous birds, shaping a basic connection in the well-established pecking order.

Grown-up mosquitoes likewise assume a part in fertilization, despite the fact that their effect in this space is less critical contrasted with different pollinators like honey bees and butterflies. While benefiting from nectar, female mosquitoes coincidentally move dust from one blossom to another, helping with the preparation interaction and working with plant propagation. However not their essential capability, this accidental fertilization can add to the biodiversity and soundness of plant networks.

Besides, mosquitoes, as different bugs, add to the general biodiversity of environments. The incredible variety of mosquito species enriches and diversifies ecosystems worldwide. Every species involves a particular biological specialty, adjusting to various natural surroundings and ecological circumstances. This variety not just guarantees the endurance of different mosquito species yet in addition gives a powerful and versatile environment.

However, it is essential to acknowledge that female mosquitoes, in particular, are well-known for their role as disease carriers, transferring pathogens that cause illnesses in both animals and humans. While we should recognize this part of their science, it is essential to find some kind of harmony between grasping their biological significance and tending to the general wellbeing concerns related with their sickness transmission abilities.

Malaria, dengue fever, the Zika virus, chikungunya, the West Nile virus, and many others are spread by mosquitoes. For egg development, female mosquitoes require a blood meal, during which they can acquire pathogens that cause disease from infected hosts. In this manner, when they feed on another host, they can communicate these microorganisms, bringing about the spread of sicknesses.

The unique feeding behavior and biological adaptations of mosquitoes are primarily responsible for their capacity to transmit diseases. Their fragile mouthparts are intended to puncture the skin of hosts, permitting them to get to veins and get a blood dinner. During this interaction, spit is infused into the host to forestall blood thickening and work with continuous taking care of. Sadly, this spit might contain illness causing microorganisms, which can be sent to the host, prompting contamination and sickness.

For public health efforts to prevent and control diseases transmitted by mosquitoes, it is essential to comprehend the disease vectoring function of mosquitoes. A variety of strategies are used to lessen the impact of these diseases, including community education, mosquito control, and surveillance.

Mosquito control programs expect to diminish mosquito populaces and breaking point their connections with people. Insecticide use, larviciding to kill mosquito larvae in breeding grounds, and adult mosquito control methods like fogging and trapping may be part of these programs. Moreover, eliminating or treating stale water sources that act as favorable places for mosquitoes is urgent to intrude on their life cycle.

Local area schooling and public mindfulness crusades assume a crucial part in counteraction endeavors. By understanding the environment of mosquitoes and the sicknesses they convey, people can go to proactive lengths to safeguard themselves and their networks. These actions might incorporate utilizing bug anti-agents, wearing defensive apparel, and killing mosquito rearing destinations around homes.

While the biological significance of mosquitoes ought not be eclipsed by their job as illness vectors, it is important to figure out some kind of harmony between protecting environment elements and defending general wellbeing. Proceeded with exploration, observation, and cooperation between scientists, entomologists, and general wellbeing experts are critical for figuring out the mind-boggling interaction between mosquitoes, microbes, and the climate.

Factors Contributing to the Proliferation of Mosquitoes

The proliferation of mosquitoes, those pesky insects that seem to buzz around us, can be attributed to various factors, with climate change and urbanization playing prominent roles. These factors have created favorable conditions for mosquito breeding and survival, increasing mosquito populations and their potential to transmit diseases. Understanding these contributing factors is crucial for implementing effective strategies to control mosquito populations and mitigate the associated risks.

One of the primary factors driving the proliferation of mosquitoes is climate change. As global temperatures rise, mosquitoes expand their geographic range and thrive in previously unsuitable areas. Warmer temperatures accelerate their reproductive cycles, resulting in more frequent breeding and larger populations. In addition, extended warm seasons provide mosquitoes with a longer window for feeding and reproduction, further fueling their proliferation.

Changes in precipitation patterns also influence mosquito populations. Increased rainfall can create more breeding sites, as mosquitoes require stagnant water for their larvae to develop. Heavy rainfall events and flooding can lead to the formation of temporary water bodies, such as puddles and pools, providing ample opportunities for mosquito breeding. Conversely, periods of drought followed by sudden rainfall can create ideal conditions for mosquito hatching, as eggs in dry areas can quickly hatch when exposed to water.

Urbanization is another significant factor contributing to the proliferation of mosquitoes. As cities expand and urban areas encroach upon natural habitats, mosquitoes find new environments suitable for breeding. Urban landscapes provide abundant artificial containers, such as discarded tires, flowerpots, and construction sites, which collect water and serve as ideal breeding grounds. Additionally, human hosts and an uninterrupted supply of blood meals contribute to the sustained growth of mosquito populations in urban areas.

Urbanization also alters local microclimates, creating warmer, humid conditions that favor mosquito survival and reproduction. The "urban heat island" effect, characterized by higher temperatures in urban areas than surrounding rural regions, creates microenvironments conducive to mosquito breeding and development. The abundance of impervious surfaces, such as concrete and asphalt, exacerbates the heat island effect by retaining heat and limiting natural cooling processes.

Furthermore, urbanization disrupts natural ecosystems and reduces biodiversity, which can indirectly contribute to mosquito proliferation. Healthy ecosystems typically include predators, such as bats, birds, and dragonflies, which feed on mosquitoes and help regulate their populations. However, urban development often leads to the destruction of natural habitats and the loss of these natural predators, allowing mosquito populations to flourish unchecked.

Human behavior and socioeconomic factors also play a role in mosquito proliferation. Inadequate waste management and the improper disposal of containers can create breeding sites for mosquitoes. The need for more awareness and education about mosquito-borne diseases and prevention measures can further exacerbate the problem. Socioeconomic disparities can contribute to the persistence of mosquito-friendly environments, as low-income communities may have limited access to mosquito control and prevention resources.

Addressing the factors contributing to the proliferation of mosquitoes requires a multi-faceted approach. Effective mosquito control and prevention strategies should include targeted interventions such as source reduction, insecticide application, and community engagement. Source reduction focuses on eliminating or modifying mosquito breeding sites, such as removing standing water and properly managing water storage containers. Insecticide application may be necessary in specific situations. Still, it should be applied judiciously and follow public health guidelines to minimize environmental and non-target organisms' adverse impacts.

Public awareness campaigns and education programs are crucial in promoting behavior change and empowering individuals to take proactive measures to prevent mosquito bites and reduce mosquito breeding. These efforts should emphasize the importance of using insect repellents, wearing protective clothing, and keeping living environments clean and free from potential breeding sites.

Climate change and urbanization have significantly contributed to the proliferation of mosquitoes. The warming temperatures, altered precipitation patterns, and modified microclimates associated with climate change create favorable conditions for mosquito survival and reproduction. Urbanization, by creating artificial breeding sites and disrupting natural ecosystems, further facilitates mosquito proliferation. Combating the proliferation of mosquitoes requires a comprehensive approach that considers environmental, socioeconomic, and public health factors. By addressing these contributing factors and implementing effective prevention and control measures, we can reduce the risks associated with mosquito-borne diseases and ensure a healthier and safer environment for all.

CHAPTER 2
Unmasking West Nile Virus: The Silent Intruder

It is essential to shed light on the West Nile virus's origins, trace its history of discovery and initial outbreaks, and investigate its subsequent global spread in order to fully comprehend its significance as a prominent disease transmitted by mosquitoes. This information not just assists us with grasping the effect of the infection on human wellbeing yet in addition features the requirement for progressing exploration, counteraction, and control measures.

The West Nile virus got its start in Uganda's West Nile district in the 1930s, which is where it got its name. Researchers recognized the infection in a lady's blood with a gentle febrile disease, denoting the underlying acknowledgment of this beforehand obscure microorganism. Around then, the clinical meaning of the infection stayed dark, and its effect on general wellbeing went to a great extent inconspicuous.

The West Nile virus remained relatively unknown for several decades following its discovery, with sporadic outbreaks reported in various regions of Africa, the Middle East, and Europe. It was mostly thought to be an endemic disease because it only caused mild febrile illness in humans and didn't kill a lot of birds.

In the summer of 1999, the West Nile virus reached a turning point in its history. New York City saw a rise in severe neurological cases, which drew the attention of scientists and public health officials alike. This episode denoted the main acknowledgment of the West Nile infection in the Western Half of the globe. It marked the beginning of a new era in our comprehension of the virus's potential effects.

Examination concerning the flare-up uncovered that the infection had likely been acquainted with New York City by bringing in contaminated birds, predominantly through the exchange of tainted fancy birds. The Culex species of mosquito, which are renowned for their preference for birds as their hosts, played a crucial role in the virus's spread from infected birds to humans and other animals. The outbreak quickly spread, infecting humans, horses, and other susceptible species and resulting in illness and death.

The development of the West Nile infection in the US provoked elevated reconnaissance and exploration endeavors. Obviously the infection was not restricted to Africa, the Center East, and Europe. In any case, it could set up a good foundation for itself in new domains. Resulting examinations uncovered that the infection had likely been coursing undetected in different locales before its rise in New York City.

Since first experience with the US, West Nile infection has spread across the mainland, influencing people, birds, and different creatures. The virus is transmitted between infected birds and susceptible hosts by mosquitoes, the primary vector. The virus has shown remarkable adaptability to various ecological settings. It has become endemic in numerous areas of North America.

The worldwide spread of the West Nile infection has been worked with by movement, exchange, and environmental change. Tainted people can unconsciously ship the infection to new districts, where neighborhood mosquitoes can in this way get and communicate the infection. Additionally, the virus can spread to previously uninfected regions through the migratory or trade movements of infected birds.

Environmental change has additionally impacted the dissemination and transmission elements of the West Nile infection. Climbing temperatures, modified precipitation examples, and changes in environmental circumstances can affect the overflow and circulation of mosquitoes and the host populaces on which they depend. These progressions can set out new open doors for the infection to spread to districts where it was beforehand missing or to set up a good foundation for itself all the more conspicuously in regions where it as of now exists.

In humans, West Nile virus infections are typically mild or asymptomatic; however, severe neurological complications can occur in some instances. These serious cases can prompt long haul medical problems and even demise. The effect of the infection on general wellbeing and its true capacity for additional spread and rise highlights the significance of continuous reconnaissance, examination, and general wellbeing intercessions.

The beginnings and history of the West Nile infection feature its change from an obscure microbe in Uganda to a universally perceived and effective mosquito-borne illness. The virus's potential for severe illness and death was made clear by the initial outbreaks in the United States, which served as a wake-up call. The virus's subsequent global spread demonstrates the significance of ongoing surveillance, research, and control measures. By understanding the beginnings and history of the West Nile infection, we can more readily value the direness of tending to this quiet gatecrasher and safeguarding human and creature wellbeing.

The Biology of West Nile Virus and Its Transmission Cycle

To grasp the effect of the West Nile virus as a mosquito-borne sickness, it is fundamental to dig into its science and comprehend its perplexing transmission cycle between mosquitoes, birds, and people. By unwinding the logical subtleties, we gain essential knowledge about how this infection spreads, and its capacity to cause sickness.

West Nile infection has a place with the Flavivirus variety and is a solitary abandoned RNA infection. Its hereditary material encodes proteins that empower the disease to recreate and connect with cells. The virus's genetic material is protected by a lipid envelope containing various proteins that make it easier for the virus to enter host cells.

There are two primary hosts in the West Nile virus transmission cycle: mosquitoes and birds. Mosquitoes are the important vectors, while birds act as the repository. The process starts when a mosquito becomes tainted by benefiting from a contaminated bird. The infection enters the mosquito's midgut, where it repeats and spreads to different tissues.

When the infection arrives at an adequate level in the mosquito's body, it tends to be sent to different hosts during resulting blood feasts. The virus is injected into the bloodstream of a susceptible bird when an infected mosquito bites it. The infection can reproduce inside the bird and arrive at significant levels, permitting it to taint different mosquitoes that feed on the bird.

The virus's survival and amplification in nature depend on this transmission cycle between birds and mosquitoes. Certain species of mosquito, especially those belonging to the genus Culex, strongly prefer bird hosts. These mosquitoes can benefit from contaminated birds, get the infection, and send it to other defenseless birds during the resulting blood feasts.

Even though birds are the primary West Nile virus hosts, infected mosquito bites can infect humans and other animals. Humans and horses are regarded as incidental hosts because they do not produce sufficient virus in their bloodstream to effectively infect mosquitoes. However, the virus may spread to other susceptible hosts if a mosquito eats an infected horse or human.

The transmission of West Nile infection from mosquitoes to people or different creatures happens through the infusion of contaminated mosquito spit while taking care. When the infection enters the host's circulatory system, it can course all through the body, possibly prompting disease.

It's important to remember that not everyone with West Nile virus has symptoms. Most diseases are asymptomatic, meaning the remaining parts are uninformed about the contamination. Be that as it may, roughly 20% of tainted people foster West Nile fever, a mild disease portrayed by the side effects, for example, fever, migraine, body hurts, and weakness. The virus can cause severe neurological disorders like encephalitis or meningitis in about 1 in 150 infections, which can result in long-term complications or even death.

The transmission elements of West Nile infection are affected by different variables. The virus's intensity and geographic distribution are all influenced by mosquito populations, bird migration patterns, and ecological conditions. Mosquitoes flourish in warm and muggy conditions, and their overflow is impacted by variables like temperature, precipitation, and the accessibility of reasonable rearing locales.

West Nile virus is highly contagious to birds, particularly those of the corvid family (crows, ravens, and jays). They can hold onto elevated degrees of the infection and act as intensifying hosts, adding to its spread inside mosquito populations. The virus can travel great distances by migrating birds, reaching new regions, and potentially spreading to susceptible people.

The disease's complexity is exemplified by how humans, birds, and mosquitoes interact in the West Nile virus transmission cycle. It is urgent to Grasp this cycle.

For executing powerful counteraction and control procedures, mosquito control measures, like the end of rearing destinations and designated bug spray application, can assist with diminishing mosquito populations and intruding on the transmission cycle. General wellbeing endeavors additionally center around surveillance and early identification of the infection, as well as state-funded training to advance individual defensive measures like utilizing mosquito anti-agents and wearing a defensive dress.

The biology of West Nile virus involves a human, bird, and mosquito transmission cycle. Mosquitoes get the infection by benefiting from tainted birds. Like this, they communicate it to other vulnerable hosts during blood feasts. While birds act as essential hosts, people, and creatures can become accidental hosts whenever nibbled by tainted mosquitoes. Understanding West Nile infection's multifaceted science and transmission pattern is fundamental for executing exciting anticipation and control measures to alleviate its effect on human and creature wellbeing.

Clinical Manifestations, Diagnosis, and Treatment of West Nile Virus Infection

West Nile Virus, a mosquito-borne microbe, can cause a scope of clinical signs in people, changing from gentle influenza like side effects to serious neurological entanglements. It is essential to have a solid understanding of the clinical aspects of West Nile virus infection for prompt diagnosis, appropriate treatment, and management.

Clinical indications of West Nile infection contamination can be ordered into three essential structures: asymptomatic contamination, West Nile fever, and neuroinvasive infection. About 70% to 80% of people who are infected with the virus don't show any symptoms and are referred to as asymptomatic carriers. They may unwittingly act as repositories for the infection, adding to its transmission.

West Nile fever is the milder form of the disease, and its symptoms are similar to those of the flu. Fever, headache, muscle and joint pain, fatigue, and occasionally a skin rash are all common signs. While most people with West Nile fever recover completely, some may endure weeks or months of weakness and fatigue.

A neuroinvasive disease that affects the central nervous system is the manifestation of West Nile virus that is the most severe. This form of the disease can result in severe neurological complications like encephalitis, meningitis, and acute flaccid paralysis, despite the fact that it is relatively uncommon. Meningitis is characterized by inflammation of the membranes that surround the brain and spinal cord, whereas encephalitis is characterized by inflammation of the brain. Intense limp loss of motion is described by unexpected shortcoming or loss of motion of appendages.

The neuroinvasive sickness can bring about numerous side effects, including high fever, extreme migraine, neck solidness, muscle shortcoming or loss of motion, confusion, seizures, quakes, and even unconsciousness. Long-term neurological impairments, such as muscle weakness, difficulty with balance and coordination, and cognitive deficits, may result from these symptoms, which range in severity.

The analysis of West Nile infection disease includes a few lab tests. A blood or cerebrospinal liquid (CSF) test might be gotten for examination in thought cases. The diagnosis can be confirmed through the detection of viral genetic material (RNA) or specific antibodies against the virus. Typically, antibodies produced by the immune system in response to the virus are detected through serological tests like enzyme-linked immunosorbent assays (ELISA). Polymerase chain response (PCR) tests are utilized to recognize the infection's hereditary material.

It is critical to take note of that the clinical show of West Nile infection contamination can cover with other mosquito-borne ailments and viral diseases, making precise conclusion testing. To make a definitive diagnosis, healthcare providers must take into account the patient's symptoms, epidemiological factors, and laboratory results.

There is no specific antiviral treatment for West Nile virus infection at this time. The patient's symptoms and supportive care are the primary focuses of management. Analgesics like acetaminophen (paracetamol) can ease fever, migraine, and muscle torment. Bed rest, hydration, and difficulty observing are fundamental for strong consideration.

Hospitalization and serious clinical administration might be expected for patients with extreme neurological complexities. Controlling seizures, reducing intracranial pressure, supporting the respiratory system, and managing other symptoms are all examples of this. In some cases, patients might require restoration administrations to help their recuperation and address any drawn out impedances.

Counteraction assumes a critical part in relieving the effect of West Nile infection contamination. General wellbeing endeavors center around mosquito control measures to diminish mosquito populaces and forestall chomps. This includes avoiding outdoor activities, using insect repellents, eliminating breeding sites in standing water, and wearing protective clothing.

During top mosquito action periods. Public education campaigns also raise public awareness of the West Nile virus, how it spreads, and how to prevent it.

Furthermore, endeavors are in progress to foster immunizations against the West Nile infection. A few exploratory immunizations have shown guarantee in preclinical and early clinical preliminaries. However, before widespread implementation can occur, additional research and development are required.

Asymptomatic cases of West Nile virus infection can be accompanied by mild flu-like symptoms or severe neurological complications. The patient's symptoms and epidemiological factors are taken into account when performing laboratory tests for an accurate diagnosis. Treatment principally includes steady consideration, tending to side effects, and overseeing intricacies. It is essential to prevent infection by controlling mosquitoes and educating the public. The management of West Nile virus infection in the future looks promising thanks to ongoing efforts in research and the development of vaccines.

Impact of West Nile Virus on Public Health, Economics, and Affected Communities

Beyond its clinical manifestations, the West Nile virus significantly affects the economy, public health, and communities. As the infection proceeds to spread and cause flare-ups, understanding its more extensive effect is fundamental for carrying out successful counteraction systems and offering essential help to those impacted.

In the face of West Nile virus outbreaks, public health is a primary concern. The infection represents a critical danger to human wellbeing, with possible extreme neurological entanglements and even demise. Neuroinvasive sickness can considerably trouble medical care frameworks, requiring particular clinical consideration, hospitalization, and recovery administrations. The expenses related to diagnosing, treating, and overseeing West Nile infection cases can strain medical care assets.

Additionally, it is essential to consider the psychological effects of West Nile virus outbreaks. The trepidation and tension encompassing the potential for contamination can create a feeling of disquiet inside networks. The vulnerability of the sickness' course, especially in severe cases, can produce extra pressure and worry for people and their friends and family. General well-being endeavors should consider tending to these mental perspectives and offering proper help and guiding administrations to those impacted.

The economic effect of the West Nile infection is multi-layered. The virus can harm tourism, outdoor recreation, and other businesses that depend on the outdoors in areas with outbreaks. Worries about the gamble of mosquito nibbles might prompt a decrease in open-air occasions, influencing nearby organizations and economies. Moreover, the expenses related to mosquito control programs, observation endeavors, and general wellbeing efforts can put a monetary weight on nearby and provincial specialists.

The farming area can likewise experience because of the effect of the West Nile infection. Numerous domestic and wild bird species are susceptible to disease by the virus. The poultry and bird-related industries can be affected by outbreaks among avian populations, which can result in bird deaths. Additionally, birds act as the virus's amplifying hosts, facilitating its spread to mosquitoes and raising the likelihood that humans will become infected. Agricultural practices and efforts to protect wildlife may be disrupted due to this interaction between human populations, mosquitoes, and avian populations.

West Nile virus outbreaks' social and economic effects frequently occur in communities directly impacted. Severe cases and fatalities can prompt a feeling of misfortune and misery inside networks. Long-term care for people with neurological problems can be emotionally and financially draining for families. Furthermore, the weight of mosquito control measures, like the end of reproducing locales and insect poison application, can fall lopsidedly on distraught networks with restricted assets.

West Nile virus may pose a more significant threat to vulnerable populations, such as the elderly and those with preexisting health conditions, who may be more susceptible to severe illness and complications. Financial differences can additionally worsen the effect of the infection, as hindered networks might confront boundaries in getting to medical care administrations, mosquito control measures, and training about preventive measures. It is essential to address these disparities to ensure equitable health outcomes and efficient prevention strategies.

Community involvement and education are necessary to lessen the West Nile virus's effects. General well-being specialists should give exact and ideal data about the infection, its transmission, and preventive measures to engage people and networks to safeguard themselves. Implementing integrated vector management strategies and fostering a collective response to the virus require collaborative efforts between public health agencies, local authorities, community organizations, and residents.

Moreover, exploration and observation endeavors are essential for grasping the study of disease transmission of the West Nile infection, checking its spread, and distinguishing potential gamble factors. Public health policies and guidelines are based on this information, making creating targeted interventions possible.

The effect of the West Nile infection reaches out past its clinical signs, influencing general well-being, financial matters, and impacted networks. Healthcare systems can be strained, local economies can be disrupted, and outbreaks can cause psychological distress.

Weak populaces might confront unbalanced loads. However, in the face of West Nile virus outbreaks, proactive public health measures, community engagement, and targeted interventions can assist in minimizing the impact and fostering resilience.

CHAPTER 3
Battling Mosquito-Borne Diseases: Prevention and Control

Preventing and Controlling Mosquito-Borne Diseases, Including West Nile Virus

Mosquito-borne illnesses, including the West Nile infection, altogether compromise general well-being. Forestalling and controlling these sicknesses requires a thorough and incorporated approach that objectives mosquitoes and human behavior. We can reduce the number of mosquitoes in a community, break the cycle of disease transmission, and shield communities from the devastating effects of diseases spread by mosquitoes by implementing various strategies.

1. Mosquito Surveillance and Monitoring:

Surveillance and monitoring of mosquito populations are crucial for understanding their distribution, abundance, and infection rates. By tracking mosquito activity, public health authorities can identify areas at high risk for disease transmission, implement targeted control measures, and provide timely warnings to the public. Surveillance also helps identify emerging mosquito-borne diseases and detect changes in mosquito behavior or insecticide resistance.

2. Source Reduction:

Source reduction aims to eliminate or modify mosquito breeding sites to reduce mosquito populations. This involves identifying and removing or treating stagnant water sources, such as discarded tires, containers, gutters, and flowerpots, where mosquitoes lay their eggs. Regular inspection and maintenance of water storage containers, proper drainage of standing water, and effective waste management practices are essential in preventing mosquito breeding and minimizing their presence in communities.

3. Larviciding:

Larviciding involves the targeted application of larvicides to kill mosquito larvae in their breeding sites. Larvicides are chemicals or biological agents that disrupt the development of mosquito larvae, preventing them from reaching adulthood. This strategy is particularly effective in controlling mosquito populations in areas with persistent breeding sites that cannot be eliminated, or other control methods are not feasible.

4. Insecticide Application:

Insecticide application is essential in controlling adult mosquito populations and interrupting disease transmission. This can be done through space spraying or fogging in areas with high mosquito activity or disease outbreaks. Insecticides are applied as ultra-low volume (ULV) sprays, targeting flying mosquitoes. It is crucial to use insecticides that are effective against the specific mosquito species of concern and to adhere to the recommended dosage and application guidelines to minimize environmental impact and ensure public safety.

5. Personal Protection Measures:

Personal protection measures are crucial in preventing mosquito bites and reducing the risk of mosquito-borne diseases. On exposed skin and clothing, individuals should be encouraged to use mosquito repellents containing EPA-registered active ingredients, such as DEET, picaridin, or IR3535. Wearing long-sleeved shirts, long pants, and socks can provide additional protection. Additionally, using bed nets treated with insecticides, particularly in areas with high malaria transmission, can protect individuals while sleeping.

6. Community Education and Awareness:

Community education and awareness campaigns are essential for promoting behavioral changes and fostering a collective effort in mosquito control. Providing accurate information about mosquito-borne diseases, their transmission, and prevention strategies can empower individuals to take proactive measures to protect themselves and their communities. Educational initiatives should target schools, healthcare facilities, community centers, and public spaces, utilizing various communication channels, including social media, pamphlets, and workshops, to disseminate information effectively.

7. Integrated Vector Management:

Integrated Vector Management (IVM) is a comprehensive approach that combines various strategies to control mosquito populations and prevent mosquito-borne diseases. IVM focuses on ecological, biological, and chemical control methods, community participation, and sustainable practices. It considers local environmental conditions, mosquito species, and the socioeconomic context of the affected communities. IVM provides a holistic and practical approach to mosquito-borne disease prevention and control by integrating different control measures and promoting community involvement.

8. Vector-Resistant Housing:

In areas with

With high mosquito-borne disease transmission, building houses with protective measures can reduce human-mosquito contact. Simple interventions, such as window screens, air conditioning, and sealing gaps and openings in homes, can prevent mosquitoes from entering indoor spaces and biting individuals. Vector-resistant housing strategies are fundamental in regions with endemic diseases like malaria, dengue, and the West Nile virus.

9. Biological Control:

Biological control methods involve using natural enemies of mosquitoes to reduce their populations. This can include the introduction of larvivorous fish, such as Gambusia affinis (mosquito fish), into water bodies to consume mosquito larvae. Biological control agents, such as bacteria (e.g., Bacillus thuringiensis israelensis) or nematodes, can target mosquito larvae while minimizing harm to non-target organisms and the environment.

10. Research and Innovation:

Continued research and innovation are vital for advancing mosquito-borne disease prevention and control strategies. This includes developing new insecticides, exploring genetic modification techniques to reduce mosquito populations, and discovering novel approaches to disrupt disease transmission cycles. Additionally, surveillance and research provide essential data on mosquito behavior, disease prevalence, and emerging threats, enabling public health authorities to adapt prevention and control strategies accordingly.

Preventing and controlling mosquito-borne diseases, including West Nile virus, require a multi-faceted approach that targets both mosquitoes and human behavior. Through surveillance, source reduction, larviciding, insecticide application, personal protection measures, community education, and integrated vector management, we can effectively reduce mosquito populations, interrupt disease transmission cycles, and protect communities from the devastating impact of mosquito-borne illnesses. Continued research and innovation are essential in refining and developing new strategies to combat these diseases and safeguard public health.

Personal Protective Measures for Mosquito-Borne Diseases

Personal protective measures are crucial in preventing mosquito bites and reducing the risk of mosquito-borne diseases. By adopting simple yet effective strategies such as using insect repellents, wearing protective clothing, and utilizing bed nets, individuals can shield themselves from mosquito vectors and their potential health risks.

1. Insect Repellents:

Insect repellents are a cornerstone of personal protection against mosquitoes. They work by creating a barrier that deters mosquitoes from landing and biting. The most commonly used active ingredients in repellents include DEET (N, N-diethyl-meta-toluamide), picaridin (KBR 3023), IR3535 (3-[N-Butyl-N-acetyl]-amino propionic acid ethyl ester), and oil of lemon eucalyptus (OLE). These repellents are registered with the Environmental

Protection Agency (EPA) and have been proven effective in repelling mosquitoes.

When using insect repellents, following the instructions on the product label is essential. Apply the repellent evenly to exposed skin, avoiding areas near the eyes, mouth, and open wounds. For application to the face, spray the repellent onto the hands and then carefully apply it. It is advisable to reapply repellents as directed, particularly if spending prolonged periods outdoors or engaging in activities that may cause excessive sweating or water exposure. After returning indoors, wash treated skin with soap and water.

2. Protective Clothing:

Wearing protective clothing can provide an additional physical barrier against mosquito bites. When spending time outdoors, particularly during peak mosquito activity periods, individuals should opt for loose-fitting, long-sleeved shirts, long pants, and socks. Mosquitoes have difficulty penetrating lightweight, loose-fitting clothing, reducing the likelihood of skin contact. Light-colored clothing is recommended, as mosquitoes are often attracted to dark colors.

For added protection, clothing treated with insecticides, such as permethrin, can be used. Permethrin-treated clothing remains effective even after multiple washes. It can provide long-lasting protection against mosquitoes and other biting insects. It is important to note that permethrin should not be applied directly to the skin but to clothing items according to the product instructions.

3. Bed Nets:

Bed nets are a valuable defense against mosquitoes, particularly those active during sleeping hours. Bed nets create a physical barrier between individuals and mosquitoes, reducing the risk of bites and exposure to mosquito-borne diseases such as malaria, dengue, and West Nile. Long-lasting insecticidal nets (LLINs) are impregnated with insecticides that repel and kill mosquitoes, offering extended protection.

When using bed nets, it is essential to properly hang and maintain them. Ensure the net is tucked securely under the mattress or sleeping surface to prevent mosquitoes from entering. Repair any holes or tears in the net promptly to maintain its effectiveness. Sleeping under a bed net, particularly in regions with high mosquito-borne disease transmission, is vital for vulnerable populations such as young children and pregnant women.

4. Integrated Personal Protection:

Utilizing a combination of personal protective measures provides a comprehensive defense against mosquito-borne diseases. In areas where mosquitoes are prevalent, individuals can optimize protection by using insect repellents, wearing protective clothing, and sleeping under bed nets simultaneously. This integrated approach offers multiple layers of defense and significantly reduces the likelihood of mosquito bites.

5. Community Education and Engagement:

Promoting community education and engagement is crucial for successfully adopting personal protective measures. Public health authorities, community leaders, and healthcare professionals are pivotal in raising awareness about mosquito-borne diseases and the importance of personal protection. Educational initiatives can include distributing.

Informational materials, organizing workshops, and using social media platforms to share knowledge and reinforce preventive measures.

Additionally, providing access to affordable and effective personal protective measures is essential. Governments, non-governmental organizations, and health agencies should strive to ensure that insect repellents, protective clothing, and bed nets are accessible to all, especially in areas where mosquito-borne diseases are prevalent. This includes addressing economic barriers, implementing distribution programs, and collaborating with local communities to prioritize and address their specific needs.

Personal protective measures are vital to reducing the risk of mosquito-borne diseases. By utilizing insect repellents, wearing protective clothing, and sleeping under bed nets, individuals can create practical barriers against mosquito vectors. Community education and engagement are vital in promoting the adoption of these measures and ensuring their accessibility. Combining personal protective measures with other mosquito control strategies can create a comprehensive defense against mosquito-borne diseases and protect our health and well-being.

Community-Based Interventions for Mosquito Control and Public Awareness

Community-based interventions play a crucial role in combating mosquito-borne diseases by involving the collective efforts of individuals, local organizations, and public health authorities. Through mosquito control programs, vector surveillance, and public awareness campaigns, communities can take proactive measures to reduce mosquito populations, prevent disease transmission, and promote a culture of prevention and awareness.

1. Mosquito Control Programs:

Mosquito control programs are community-based initiatives that aim to reduce mosquito populations and minimize the risk of disease transmission. These programs typically involve a combination of strategies such as source reduction, larviciding, and insecticide application to target mosquito breeding sites and adult populations. Local authorities often implement them in collaboration with public health agencies and community stakeholders.

Source reduction is critical to mosquito control programs, focusing on eliminating or modifying mosquito breeding sites. Community involvement is essential to identifying and addressing potential breeding sites in and around residential areas, parks, and public spaces. This may include removing stagnant water sources, cleaning gutters, and ensuring proper drainage. By reducing breeding sites, communities can significantly impact mosquito populations and disease transmission.

Larviciding, the targeted application of larvicides to mosquito breeding sites, is another strategy employed in mosquito control programs. These larvicides disrupt mosquito development, preventing larvae from reaching adulthood. Community participation can enhance larviciding efforts by reporting potential breeding sites and actively supporting larvicide application in stormwater drains, water storage containers, and other standing water sources.

Insecticide application, such as space spraying or fogging, is often used in response to increased mosquito activity or disease outbreaks. This approach targets adult mosquitoes and aims to reduce their populations. Community-based mosquito control programs can coordinate these efforts, ensuring that insecticide application is carried out effectively and safely, adhering to recommended guidelines and considering environmental impact.

2. Vector Surveillance:

Vector surveillance is a fundamental component of community-based interventions for mosquito-borne diseases. It involves monitoring mosquito populations, identifying species, and assessing their infection rates.

Regular surveillance allows public health authorities to obtain critical data on mosquito abundance, distribution, and disease prevalence. This information helps inform targeted control measures and identify high-risk areas for disease transmission.

Community participation in vector surveillance is invaluable. Engaging community members as citizen scientists can involve them in monitoring mosquito populations, reporting mosquito activity, and assisting with data collection. This collaborative approach provides valuable data, empowers individuals to actively contribute to disease prevention efforts, and fosters a sense of ownership and responsibility within the community.

3. Public Awareness Campaigns:

Public awareness campaigns are essential in promoting a culture of prevention and empowering individuals to protect themselves from mosquito-borne diseases. These campaigns aim to educate communities about the risks associated with mosquito bites, the importance of personal protective measures, and the role of community-based interventions.

Public health authorities and local organizations can develop comprehensive awareness campaigns that utilize various communication channels, including television, radio, social media, and community workshops. These campaigns should provide accurate information on mosquito-borne diseases, their transmission, and preventive measures such as using insect repellents, wearing protective clothing, and eliminating breeding sites.

Engaging community leaders, schools, healthcare providers, and local organizations is crucial in disseminating information effectively and fostering behavior change. Public awareness campaigns can involve workshops, interactive educational sessions, and distribution of informational materials such as brochures, posters, and pamphlets. These materials should be culturally sensitive, accessible, and available in multiple languages to reach diverse communities.

Furthermore, public awareness campaigns can be tailored to address specific local challenges and concerns. For example, in areas with a high prevalence of dengue fever, campaigns may focus on

Water storage practices and educating individuals on the importance of covering or treating water containers. By addressing local contexts and engaging the community, these campaigns have the potential to evoke meaningful behavioral changes and create lasting impact.

Community-based interventions are vital in combating mosquito-borne diseases. Mosquito control programs, vector surveillance, and public awareness campaigns empower communities to actively participate in disease prevention efforts. By implementing these interventions, communities can reduce mosquito populations, prevent disease transmission, and promote a culture of prevention and awareness. Engaging community members, utilizing local resources, and tailoring interventions to address specific challenges are vital to the success of these community-based efforts.

The Role of Technology and Innovation in Mosquito Control

Technology and innovation have revolutionized mosquito control, offering new avenues for combating mosquito-borne diseases. From genetically modified mosquitoes to novel insecticides, these advancements can potentially transform how we approach mosquito control, reducing populations and preventing disease transmission.

1. Genetically Modified Mosquitoes:

Genetically modified mosquitoes (GMMs) have emerged as promising mosquito control tools. One innovative approach involves the release of male mosquitoes carrying an altered gene that causes offspring to die before adulthood. These male mosquitoes, known as the sterile insect technique (SIT), mate with wild females, reducing the overall mosquito population over time.

Another approach involves the release of genetically modified male mosquitoes carrying a gene that causes female offspring to be sterile. The incompatible insect technique (IIT) aims to reduce mosquito populations by decreasing the number of viable offspring produced.

These innovative strategies offer the potential to significantly reduce mosquito populations in a targeted and environmentally friendly manner. However, rigorous testing and regulatory oversight are essential to ensure the safety and efficacy of genetically modified mosquitoes before their widespread deployment.

2. Novel Insecticides:

Novel insecticides are another area of technological advancement in mosquito control. Researchers are continually exploring new compounds and formulations to enhance mosquito control efficacy while minimizing environmental impact and reducing the development of insecticide resistance.

One notable development is using insecticides with new modes of action that target specific biological processes in mosquitoes. These insecticides can be more selective, reducing harm to non-target organisms and decreasing the risk of resistance development. Additionally, researchers are investigating the potential of botanical extracts and natural compounds as alternatives to synthetic insecticides, offering environmentally friendly options for mosquito control.

Furthermore, innovative formulations are being developed to enhance the effectiveness and longevity of insecticides. Microencapsulation and slow-release formulations allow for the sustained release of insecticides over time, improving their persistence and reducing the frequency of reapplication. This approach enhances the efficiency of insecticide use, making it more cost-effective and reducing environmental exposure.

3. Remote Sensing and Geographic Information Systems (GIS):

Remote sensing and Geographic Information Systems (GIS) have become valuable mosquito control and surveillance tools. Satellite imagery and aerial drones can provide high-resolution data on land cover, vegetation, and water bodies, aiding in identifying potential mosquito breeding sites. This information enables targeted mosquito control interventions and resource allocation.

GIS technology allows for integrating and analyzing various data sources, such as mosquito surveillance data, environmental factors, and human population distribution. By overlaying these datasets, public health authorities can identify high-risk areas for mosquito-borne diseases and implement preventive measures accordingly. GIS-based models can also predict mosquito population dynamics and disease transmission patterns, enabling proactive interventions and timely responses to outbreaks.

4. Mosquito Trapping and Monitoring Devices:

Advancements in mosquito trapping and monitoring devices have greatly improved surveillance and control efforts. These devices employ various innovative technologies to attract and capture mosquitoes, including light traps, gravid traps, and overlaps. They can be equipped with sensors to collect data on mosquito species, abundance, and infection rates.

Mechanical traps and monitoring systems, such as mosquito surveillance networks, provide real-time information on mosquito activity and allow immediate response to mosquito population changes. This data-driven approach enhances the efficiency of mosquito control programs, enabling targeted interventions and resource optimization.

5. Data Analysis and Modeling:

Data analysis and modeling techniques are instrumental in mosquito control strategies. By harnessing large datasets, researchers can analyze mosquito population dynamics, disease prevalence, and environmental factors to gain insights into mosquito-borne disease transmission patterns.

Mathematical models, such as transmission models and population models, can simulate

The spread of mosquito-borne diseases and assess the impact of different control strategies. These models help inform decision-making, evaluate the effectiveness of interventions, and guide resource allocation in mosquito control programs.

Machine learning and artificial intelligence algorithms can also analyze complex datasets, identify patterns, and predict mosquito population trends. These tools enable more accurate forecasting, early detection of disease outbreaks, and proactive control measures.

In conclusion, technology and innovation can potentially revolutionize mosquito control efforts. Genetically modified mosquitoes, novel insecticides, remote sensing, GIS, mosquito trapping devices, and data analysis techniques offer new avenues for reducing mosquito populations and preventing disease transmission. Continued research, regulatory oversight, and collaboration between scientists, public health authorities, and communities are essential in harnessing the power of technology to effectively combat mosquito-borne diseases and protect public health.

CHAPTER 4
The Future of Mosquito-Borne Disease Management

Current Advancements in Mosquito Control and Disease Management

Advancements in mosquito control and disease management have paved the way for more effective strategies in combating mosquito-borne diseases. From novel technologies and innovative approaches to vaccines and treatment options, these advancements offer promising solutions for reducing mosquito populations and improving the management of mosquito-borne diseases.

1. Novel Technologies:

Novel technologies have revolutionized mosquito control efforts, providing more targeted and efficient approaches. One such technology is mosquito traps equipped with attractants and sensors targeting disease-carrying mosquito species. These traps are designed to capture and monitor mosquitoes in high-risk areas, providing valuable data for surveillance and control measures.

Innovative tools such as "gene drive" technology are being explored to suppress mosquito populations. Gene drive involves modifying the genetics of mosquitoes to alter their reproductive capabilities, ultimately reducing their population over time. Although still experimental, this technology shows potential for long-term mosquito control and disease prevention.

2. Insecticide-Treated Bed Nets and Indoor Residual Spraying:

Insecticide-treated bed nets (ITNs) and indoor residual spraying (IRS) have been instrumental in reducing the burden of mosquito-borne diseases, particularly malaria. ITNs are designed to create a physical barrier and contain insecticides that repel and kill mosquitoes. They have been widely distributed in high-risk areas, significantly reducing the number of mosquito bites and malaria transmission.

IRS involves the application of long-lasting insecticides on the walls and ceilings of dwellings, targeting mosquitoes that come into contact with these surfaces.

This strategy provides sustained protection against mosquitoes and has effectively reduced malaria transmission in many regions.

3. Vaccines:

The development of vaccines against mosquito-borne diseases has shown promising results in disease prevention. For example, developing a vaccine against dengue fever has advanced, offering possible protection against this widespread and severe mosquito-borne disease. Vaccines stimulate the immune system to recognize and respond to specific pathogens, preventing infection or reducing the severity of the disease.

In recent years, progress has been made in developing vaccines against other mosquito-borne diseases, such as Zika and chikungunya. While these vaccines are still under investigation and require further research, they hold promise for future disease prevention and control.

4. Treatment Options:

Efforts to improve treatment options for mosquito-borne diseases are ongoing. Antiviral drugs are being developed and tested to target specific viral infections mosquitoes transmit. These drugs aim to inhibit viral replication, alleviate symptoms, and reduce the severity of the disease. While antiviral treatments are available for some mosquito-borne diseases, such as the West Nile virus, ongoing research aims to expand treatment options for a broader range of conditions.

In the case of malaria, the widespread use of artemisinin-based combination therapies (ACTs) has been pivotal in reducing mortality rates and improving treatment outcomes. ACTs are effective against the malaria parasite, Plasmodium and have become the standard treatment for uncomplicated malaria cases.

5. Integrated Vector Management:

Integrated Vector Management (IVM) approaches encompass strategies to control mosquito populations and reduce disease transmission. This comprehensive approach involves a range of interventions, including source reduction, larviciding, insecticide application, personal protective measures, and community engagement.

IVM emphasizes tailoring interventions to local contexts and involving communities in decision-making processes. IVM offers a holistic and sustainable approach to mosquito control and disease management by integrating multiple strategies and considering environmental, social, and economic factors.

6. Data-driven Approaches:

Data collection, analysis, and modeling advancements have significantly improved mosquito control and disease management strategies.

Data-driven approaches, such as Geographic Information Systems (GIS), remote sensing, and mathematical modeling, provide valuable insights into mosquito population dynamics, disease transmission patterns, and the impact of control measures.

Integrating various data sources, including mosquito surveillance data, environmental factors, and human demographics, enables targeted interventions, resource optimization, and early detection of disease outbreaks. They also facilitate evidence-based decision-making and the evaluation of control strategies, leading to more effective disease management.

Mosquito control and disease management advancements offer new hope in combating mosquito-borne diseases. Novel technologies, such as gene drives and mosquito traps, provide targeted and innovative approaches to reducing mosquito populations. Vaccines and treatment options hold promise in disease prevention and improving patient outcomes. Integrated Vector Management and data-driven approaches enhance the efficiency and effectiveness of control strategies. Continued research, investment, and collaboration are crucial in advancing these innovations and ultimately reducing the global burden of mosquito-borne diseases.

Challenges and Opportunities in the Fight Against Mosquito-Borne Diseases

Combatting mosquito-borne diseases poses significant challenges but also presents opportunities for innovation, collaboration, and global health advancements. Various factors, including climate change, drug resistance, and the need for international cooperation, shape the landscape of mosquito-borne disease control. Understanding these challenges and seizing the opportunities they offer is crucial in our efforts to reduce the burden of these diseases

1. Climate Change:

Climate change plays a pivotal role in the spread and intensity of mosquito-borne diseases. Rising temperatures, altered precipitation patterns, and changing ecological conditions impact mosquito populations, their geographic distribution, and the length of transmission seasons. These changes create new mosquito habitats and enhance their ability to reproduce and transmit diseases.

Adapting to the challenges posed by climate change requires a multidimensional approach. This includes implementing proactive surveillance and response systems to monitor changing mosquito populations, strengthening vector control strategies in vulnerable regions, and promoting community engagement and education on climate-resilient practices. Furthermore, addressing the root causes of climate change through sustainable development and reducing greenhouse gas emissions is essential for long-term disease prevention.

2. Drug Resistance:

Drug resistance is a growing concern in the management of mosquito-borne diseases. Mosquitoes and the pathogens they transmit can develop resistance to the drugs used for prevention and treatment. For instance, the emergence of artemisinin resistance in malaria parasites has posed significant challenges to malaria control efforts.

Research and development of new drugs and treatment regimens are critical to addressing drug resistance. This involves identifying alternative antimalarial compounds and improving the efficacy of existing drugs. Additionally, implementing strategies to slow the development and spread of drug resistance, such as combination therapies and rational drug use practices, is crucial. International collaboration and coordination are vital for monitoring drug resistance trends, sharing knowledge, and ensuring that effective treatments are accessible to all.

3. Vector Control Challenges:

Vector control remains a cornerstone in combating mosquito-borne diseases. However, several challenges exist in implementing effective control measures. Mosquitoes have adapted to various control methods, such as insecticides and larvicides, leading to the development of resistance. This necessitates the ongoing research and development of new and innovative approaches to combat resistance and enhance the effectiveness of vector control strategies.

Moreover, reaching vulnerable populations, particularly those in remote and resource-limited areas, poses challenges in implementing comprehensive vector control programs. Limited access to healthcare services, inadequate infrastructure, and cultural barriers can hinder the success of interventions. Community engagement, education, and local capacity-building are essential to overcome these challenges. Empowering communities to actively participate in vector control efforts can promote sustainability and improve the overall effectiveness of interventions.

4. International Cooperation:

Mosquito-borne diseases are not confined by national borders. They require international cooperation and collaboration to effectively address the global burden. Sharing knowledge, expertise, and resources among countries is crucial in developing and implementing effective prevention and control strategies. International organizations, such as the World Health Organization (WHO) and the Centers for Disease Control and Prevention (CDC), play a vital role in facilitating coordination, providing technical guidance, and supporting capacity-building efforts.

International cooperation also extends to research and development. Collaborative efforts among scientists, institutions, and governments are essential for advancing our understanding of mosquito biology, disease transmission, and control methods. The global community can accelerate progress in combating mosquito-borne diseases by fostering partnerships, sharing data, and promoting open access to research findings.

5. Technological Innovation:

Technological advancements present unique opportunities in the fight against mosquito-borne diseases. Innovations such as genetically modified mosquitoes, novel insecticides, and digital tools for surveillance and monitoring provide new avenues for disease control. These

Technologies have the potential to revolutionize mosquito control strategies, enhance disease surveillance capabilities, and improve response times to outbreaks.

However, the responsible development and deployment of these technologies are essential. Regulatory frameworks, ethical considerations, and long-term safety assessments are necessary to ensure these innovations' effective and ethical use. Collaboration between researchers, policymakers, and communities is crucial in guiding these technologies' development, evaluation, and implementation while ensuring transparency and addressing concerns.

Combating mosquito-borne diseases is a complex challenge that requires addressing various factors. Climate change, drug resistance, vector control challenges, international cooperation, and technological innovation shape the landscape of disease control. Embracing the opportunities offered by these challenges, such as fostering global collaboration, investing in research and development, and leveraging technological advancements, is essential in reducing the burden of mosquito-borne diseases. By working together, we can overcome these challenges and strive towards a world where these diseases are effectively controlled and the health and well-being of communities are safeguarded.

The Potential of Emerging Technologies in Disease Prevention and Control

Emerging technologies have the potential to revolutionize disease prevention and control efforts, offering innovative approaches to combat mosquito-borne diseases. Gene editing and predictive modeling are two promising areas that hold tremendous promise in enhancing our ability to prevent, control, and ultimately eliminate these diseases.

1. Gene Editing:

Gene editing technologies, such as CRISPR-Cas9, have emerged as powerful tools in disease control. These technologies allow scientists to make precise modifications to the genetic material of organisms, including mosquitoes, with the potential to disrupt disease transmission cycles.

In the context of mosquito-borne diseases, gene editing offers several possibilities. One approach involves modifying the genes of mosquitoes to make them resistant to specific pathogens, effectively blocking disease transmission. For example, scientists have successfully altered the genes of Anopheles mosquitoes, the primary malaria vector, to make them resistant to the malaria parasite. This breakthrough could reduce malaria transmission in areas where these genetically modified mosquitoes are released.

Another application of gene editing is the creation of gene drive systems. Gene drive involves modifying the genetics of mosquitoes to ensure the spread of specific genetic traits through populations. This technology could reduce mosquito populations or even eradicate particular mosquito species, interrupting disease transmission. However, ethical considerations, regulatory frameworks, and careful evaluation are crucial to ensure gene drive technologies' safe and responsible use.

2. Predictive Modeling:

Predictive modeling, coupled with advanced data analytics, is transforming disease prevention and control strategies. By leveraging large datasets, including environmental, climatic, and socio-economic factors, predictive models can forecast disease transmission patterns, identify high-risk areas, and guide targeted interventions.

These models allow public health authorities to anticipate disease outbreaks, allocate resources efficiently, and implement preventive measures promptly. For example, predictive models have been successfully used to forecast the spread of dengue fever, enabling proactive vector control efforts and public health campaigns.

Furthermore, integrating real-time data, such as mosquito surveillance and climate data, enhances the accuracy and reliability of predictive models. This dynamic approach enables rapid response to changing disease dynamics and improves the effectiveness of control strategies.

3. Synergy between Technologies:

The potential synergy between gene editing and predictive modeling is fascinating. Predictive modeling can inform the design and deployment of gene editing strategies, optimizing their impact and cost-effectiveness. For example, predictive models can identify regions with high disease burden and vector abundance, guiding decisions on where to introduce genetically modified mosquitoes or other gene editing interventions.

Conversely, gene editing technologies can enhance predictive modeling by modifying mosquito traits influencing disease transmission dynamics. By incorporating genetic data into predictive models, researchers can better understand how genetic modifications in mosquito populations can affect disease transmission and predict the potential impact of gene editing interventions.

4. Ethical Considerations and Responsible Implementation:

While emerging technologies hold great promise, ethical considerations, and responsible implementation are essential. Open dialogue, stakeholder engagement, and community involvement are critical in addressing ethical concerns, ensuring transparency, and fostering trust.

Ethical considerations include:

Assessing potential risks to human health and the environment.

Understanding the long-term effects of genetic modifications.

Evaluating the social implications of implementing gene editing technologies.

Regulatory frameworks and international guidelines are vital in governing these technologies' responsible development and use, ensuring safety, equity, and informed decision-making.

Additionally, transparency in research, open access to scientific findings, and public education are crucial in building public trust and facilitating meaningful discussions on the benefits, risks, and implications of emerging technologies in disease prevention and control.

In conclusion, emerging technologies such as gene editing and predictive modeling can transform disease prevention and control strategies for mosquito-borne diseases. Gene editing can disrupt

Disease transmission cycles and reduce mosquito populations, while predictive modeling enables proactive interventions and resource optimization. The synergy between these technologies holds great promise in enhancing our ability to prevent and control mosquito-borne diseases. However, responsible implementation, regulatory oversight, and ethical considerations are imperative to ensure these technologies' safe and ethical use for the benefit of global health. By embracing emerging technologies, we can continue to push the boundaries of disease control and work towards a future where mosquito-borne diseases are effectively prevented and controlled.

CONCLUSION

In conclusion, this book has explored the multifaceted world of mosquito-borne diseases, focusing on the causes, solutions, prevention, and transmission of these illnesses. Throughout its chapters, we have delved into mosquitoes' life cycle and anatomy, examined different species and their geographical distribution, and highlighted their ecological importance and role as disease vectors. We have shed light on the origins and history of the West Nile virus, its biology, and its transmission and explored its clinical manifestations, diagnosis, and treatment options.

The book has analyzed the impact of the West Nile virus on public health, economics, and affected communities, providing insight into the far-reaching consequences of mosquito-borne diseases. We have also discussed various prevention and control strategies, including personal protective measures, community-based interventions, and the potential of technology and innovation in mosquito control.

Moreover, we have examined the challenges and opportunities in combating mosquito-borne diseases, considering climate change, drug resistance, and international cooperation. The book has emphasized the need for collaborative efforts, community engagement, and responsible implementation of emerging technologies, such as gene editing and predictive modeling, in disease prevention and control.

Throughout these discussions, it has become evident that the fight against mosquito-borne diseases requires a comprehensive and integrated approach. It necessitates the involvement of individuals, communities, healthcare providers, researchers, policymakers, and international organizations. By combining scientific advancements, technological innovation, and community-driven strategies, we can significantly reduce the burden of mosquito-borne diseases and improve global health outcomes.

This book serves as a guide, providing valuable insights, knowledge, and practical information for readers interested in understanding the complexities of mosquito-borne diseases and the measures taken to combat them. We hope the information presented in these pages will raise awareness, inspire further research, and encourage individuals and communities to take proactive steps toward prevention and control.

Ultimately, our collective efforts and commitment are crucial in mitigating the impact of mosquito-borne diseases, improving public health, and creating a world where individuals can thrive free from the threat of these illnesses. Through continued research, innovation, education, and global collaboration, we can significantly reduce the burden of mosquito-borne diseases and ensure a healthier and safer future for generations to come.